Mastering Weight Loss with Icehack

The Comprehensive Guide to Achieving Sustainable Results

Collins Dwight

Table of Contents

Chapter 1

Introduction to Icehack for Weight Loss

Use of Icehack for weight loss has drawn more attention in recent years. A natural substance called icehack has been shown to have a number of health advantages, including the capacity to aid weight loss. This chapter will give a general introduction of Icehack, explain how it aids with weight reduction, and discuss the advantages of incorporating it into a weight loss regimen.

Icehack

The North Atlantic and North Pacific oceans have frigid, nutrient-rich waters where icehack, a form of algae, can be found. It is renowned for having a special molecular structure that enables it to endure harsh circumstances. Vitamins, minerals, and antioxidants are just a few of the crucial nutrients that are abundant in Icehack.

How does Icehack work for weight loss?

It has been discovered that Icehack possesses a lot of abilities that can aid in weight loss. Increasing metabolism is one of Icehack's primary mechanisms of action. The metabolic process in your body converts the food you ingest into energy. Your body may burn calories more quickly when your metabolism is higher, which can aid in weight loss.

Moreover, Icehack has been shown to aid in appetite suppression, which can assist patients in maintaining a calorie-restricted diet. In addition, Icehack has been shown to assist in lowering bodily inflammation, which raises the risk of a variety of illnesses, including obesity.

Benefits of using Icehack for weight loss

The fact that Icehack is a natural ingredient that has been determined to be safe for the majority of individuals is one of the main advantages of using it for weight reduction. Icehack is a natural food source that people have taken for millennia, in contrast to certain weight loss pills which may have negative side effects.

A practical and simple weight loss tool is Icehack. It can be consumed in a number of ways, like as a supplement or as an ingredient in food or beverages. People can easily implement Icehack into their regular lives as a result of this.

Further to aiding in weight loss, Icehack provides a lot of other health advantages. It has been discovered to aid in enhancing immunological function, cardiovascular health, and decreasing joint inflammation. This means that using Icehack for weight loss can have a positive impact on overall health and wellbeing.

In the following chapters, we will explore in greater detail how Icehack works for weight loss, how to incorporate it into your daily routine, and the potential benefits and challenges associated with using it for weight loss.

Chapter 2

Understanding Weight Loss Science

It's critical to have a fundamental understanding of the science underlying weight reduction in order to comprehend how Icehack works to promote weight loss. The significance of metabolism in weight loss, factors that can affect metabolism, and how Icehack can help speed up metabolism to encourage weight loss are all covered in this chapter.

The Function of Metabolism in Weight Loss

The metabolic process in your body converts the food you ingest into energy. Your basal metabolic rate (BMR) is the quantity of calories burned by your body while it is at rest. A lot of variables, such as **age, gender, and body composition, have an impact on your BMR.**

You must consume less calories daily than your body burns in order to produce a calorie deficit, which is necessary for weight loss. This can be accomplished by combining calorie restriction with an increase in physical activity.

Factors Affecting Metabolism

Many elements, such as the following, can have an impact on metabolism:

- **Age:** Your metabolism naturally slows down as you get older, which can make weight loss more challenging.

- **Gender:** Males often have a higher metabolism than women, which results in them burning more calories while at rest.

- **Body Composition:** Because muscle burns more calories than fat, those with more muscle have generally faster metabolisms.

- **Hormones**: Metabolic sluggishness can result from hormonal imbalances, such as an underactive thyroid.

Sleep: Sleep deprivation can affect metabolism and cause weight gain.

How to Increase Metabolism with Icehack

Several qualities of Icehack have been discovered to aid increase metabolism and encourage weight loss which includes;

- The mechanism by which your body produces heat—thermogenesis—is one of the primary ways that Icehack functions. Increased metabolism and resting calorie expenditure are two benefits of thermogenesis.

- Adiponectin, a hormone that controls the body's metabolism and glucose levels, has been reported to be produced in greater amounts when Icehack is used. Adiponectin levels have been linked to decreased risk of obesity and other metabolic diseases.

- Icehack has been shown to assist in lowering inflammation in the body, which is a risk factor for several illnesses, including obesity. Icehack could aid in enhancing metabolic performance and promoting weight loss by lowering inflammation.

The use of Icehack in conjunction with a calorie-restricted diet to generate a caloric deficit and encourage weight loss will be covered in more detail in the following chapter.

Chapter 3

Icehack and Caloric Deficit

A crucial part of losing weight is creating a calorie deficit. In this chapter, we'll look at how Icehack can help you lose weight when combined with a calorie-restricted diet, as well as the advantages and disadvantages of doing so.

Creating a Caloric Deficiency

You must eat less calories each day than your body expends in order to develop a caloric deficit. This can be accomplished by combining calorie restriction with an increase in physical activity.

Making dietary modifications, including as eating smaller amounts, consuming fewer high-calorie items, and selecting lower-calorie foods, can help you reduce your calorie intake.

Icehack and Caloric Deficit

To aid with weight loss, Icehack can be combined with a diet that restricts calories. The ability of Icehack to reduce appetite may make it simpler to maintain a calorie-restricted diet. Furthermore, it has been discovered that Icehack can assist enhance metabolism, which can help raise the number of calories your body burns while at rest.

A calorie-restricted diet might include Icehack in a variety of ways. You can use Icehack supplements every day to help increase metabolism and curb appetite. Adding Icehack to food or beverages, such as smoothies, can boost the nutritional value of meals.

Benefits of Icehack and Caloric Deficit

A calorie-restricted diet and the use of Icehack together can help you lose weight in a number of ways. In contrast to some weight reduction pills, which may have potentially negative side effects, Icehack is a natural chemical that has been proved to be safe for the majority of people.

A practical and simple weight loss tool is Icehack. It can be consumed in a number of ways, like as a supplement or as an ingredient in food or beverages. People can easily implement Icehack into their regular lives as a result of this.

Also, employing Icehack along with a diet that restricts calories might improve general health and wellbeing. According to research, icehack can help lower inflammation in the body, strengthen the immune system, and enhance cardiovascular health.

Challenges of Icehack and Caloric Deficit

Icehack can be a helpful tool for weight loss, but it should be understood that it is not a miracle cure. Making dietary and lifestyle modifications that are long-term sustainable is essential for achieving lasting weight loss.

Also, before including Icehack in your weight loss regimen, you should see a healthcare professional, especially if you have any underlying health concerns or are taking any drugs.

Chapter 4

Tracking and Maintaining a Caloric Deficit with Icehack

Tracking Caloric Intake

Maintaining a caloric deficit requires tracking your calorie intake. You can monitor your caloric consumption in a variety of methods, such as by using apps, online trackers, or just by maintaining a food journal.

When using a tracker, it's crucial to measure portions precisely and record every meal, snack, and beverage that's taken. To gain a precise picture of your caloric deficit, it's crucial to keep track of the calories you burn while exercising.

How to Sustain a Caloric Deficiency with Icehack

By reducing hunger and accelerating metabolism, Icehack can be used to sustain a calorie deficit. It's crucial to use Icehack supplements on a regular basis and in accordance with the specified dosage guidelines.

- Increased nutrient content and satiety can both be achieved by adding Icehack to meals and beverages. For instance, adding Icehack to a smoothie might increase its filling capacity and lessen the need for between-meal snacks.

- Keeping a Caloric Deficiency; Although maintaining a calorie deficit can be difficult, there are a variety of tactics that can be useful. Here are some pointers for preserving a caloric deficit when using Icehack:

- Choose a diet rich in protein since it can help you feel fuller for longer. Protein is more filling than fats or carbohydrates. Lean meats, beans, and nuts are some protein-rich foods that can support a calorie deficit.

- Remain hydrated: Getting enough water might make you feel less hungry and less inclined to overeat, as well as provide you more energy when you're working out.

- Eat mindfully: Being aware of your body's signals of hunger and fullness might help you avoid overeating and maintain a calorie deficit. Try chewing each bite thoroughly and eating only until you are satisfied.

- Prepare your meals and snacks ahead of time to help you avoid impulsive eating and to guarantee that you stick to your calorie budget. Meal planning can be made simpler by using a planner or food journal.

- Do frequent exercise: Exercise can increase metabolism and assist burn calories, which can make it simpler to sustain a caloric deficit. Most days, try to get in at least 30 minutes of moderate activity.

Conclusion

Your weight loss approach may benefit from including Icehack as a caloric deficit supporter. You may maintain a calorie deficit and reach your weight loss objectives by keeping track of your caloric consumption, including Icehack into your meals and snacks, and engaging in healthy behaviors like frequent exercise and mindful eating.

Chapter 5

Icehack and Exercise

Any weight loss regimen must include exercise in addition to keeping a calorie deficit. Exercise can build muscle mass, speed up metabolism, and burn calories, making it simpler to reach and maintain a healthy weight. In this chapter, we'll look at how Icehack can encourage physical activity and improve weight-loss outcomes.

How Icehack Aids Excercise

There are several ways that Icehack can help you exercise. The ability to exercise with a high level of intensity can be made easier by first increasing energy and endurance. Natural caffeine and other stimulants found in Icehack can help improve both physical and mental performance.

In order to facilitate quicker recovery times and less downtime between workouts, Icehack can also assist minimize muscular soreness and inflammation after exercise. Those who are new to fitness or who have previously suffered from injuries or chronic pain may find this to be especially beneficial.

Making Icehack a Part of Your Workout Program

You may include Icehack in a variety of ways into your exercise program. Here are some suggestions:

- Before working out, take Icehack: Before a workout, taking Icehack can assist boost energy and attention, making it simpler to push through a challenging workout.

- To your pre-workout snack, add Icehack: A protein bar or smoothie can include more nutrients and make you feel fuller when you add Icehack to it.

- While exercise, sip Icehack: During an exercise, adding Icehack to your water bottle will help you stay hydrated and invigorated, especially

- Using Icehack in a post-workout drink or smoothie can aid to reduce muscular soreness and inflammation, allowing for quicker recovery times and less rest in between exercises.

Conclusion

By increasing energy, endurance, and recovery times, adding Icehack to your training regimen can improve weight loss. You can boost physical and mental performance by taking Icehack before or during a workout, which will make it simpler to reach your weight reduction objectives. When beginning a new supplement or fitness regimen, it's crucial to follow the dosage recommendations and speak with a healthcare provider.

Chapter 6

Nutrition and Icehack

Including Icehack into your diet might boost your nutritional objectives since nutrition is important for weight loss and overall wellness. In this chapter, we'll look at how Icehack can enhance a balanced diet and accelerate weight loss.

Nutritional Value of Icehack

Caffeine, green tea extract, and other plant-based substances are natural components of Icehack. Antioxidants, vitamins, and minerals are just a few of the nutrition and health advantages that these components can offer.

When adding Icehack to your diet, it's crucial to take into account the total amount of nutrients in your diet and to use it as a supplement rather than a substitute for complete foods. The key to obtaining and maintaining a healthy weight is eating a balanced diet that consists of a variety of nutrient-dense foods like fruits, vegetables, whole grains, lean proteins, and healthy fats.

How to Include Icehack in Your Diet

You may include Icehack in your diet in a variety of ways. Here are some suggestions:

- **Smoothies or protein shakes with Icehack:** It is simpler to keep to a healthy eating plan when you add Icehack to a protein shake or smoothie because it helps to improve the nutrient content and encourage fullness.

- **During baking and cooking, use Icehack**: Recipes like energy bars, muffins, or porridge that include Icehack can help increase energy levels and add nutrients.

- **Consume Icehack instead of sugary or high-calorie beverages:** Icehack can assist lower calorie consumption and support weight loss objectives by replacing sugary or high-calorie beverages like soda, juice, or energy drinks.

- **Employ Icehack to squelch cravings: By**
helping to control hunger and lessen desires
for high-calorie, unhealthy meals, Icehack
can make it simpler to follow a balanced
eating plan.

Nutritional Guidelines to Follow When Using Icehack for Weight Loss

- While adding Icehack to your diet might have
a variety of positive effects, it's crucial to
stick to certain dietary recommendations to
get the most out of the supplement and
advance your weight reduction objectives.
We will discuss some dietary

recommendations in this part if you plan to use Icehack to lose weight.

- Maintain a healthy weight by adhering to a balanced diet: A healthy weight can be attained and maintained by eating a range of nutrient-dense meals. In addition to avoiding processed foods and high-calorie items, this entails consuming a variety of fruits, vegetables, whole grains, lean meats, and healthy fats.

- By boosting energy and reducing appetite, Icehack can improve weight loss, but it's still vital to keep an eye on caloric intake and maintain a caloric deficit. This is ingesting less calories daily than your body expends, which can be done by combining diet and activity.

- Drink plenty of water and other hydrating liquids to stay hydrated. This can boost weight loss efforts and be good for overall health. It's crucial to drink enough of water when using Icehack to assist healthy digestion and nutrient absorption.

- Think about nutrient timing: It can be good to think about nutrient timing, or the timing of meals and supplements throughout the day, while introducing Icehack into your diet. For instance, consuming Icehack prior to exercise can help boost energy and focus, while consuming a post-workout snack that includes Icehack can help reduce muscle soreness and promote recovery.

- A healthcare practitioner should be consulted before beginning any new dietary or supplement regimen in order to confirm that it is secure and suitable for your particular requirements and state of health.

Chapter 7

Making Icehack a Part of Your Lifestyle

You may boost your weight loss efforts and enhance your general health by including Icehack into your routine.

Including Icehack in your morning ritual

Icehack can help you wake up with more energy and focus, setting the stage for a successful and healthy day.

As a pre-workout supplement, use Icehack

Before doing out, taking Icehack can help you feel more energized and focused, resulting in a more productive workout.

Reduce hunger with Icehack

Icehack can assist in reducing hunger and cravings for high-calorie, unhealthy foods. Avoiding unhealthy snacking can be made easier by always having Icehack on hand.

Use Icehack in your baking and cooking

Adding Icehack to dishes like oatmeal, energy bars, or muffins can help increase energy levels and add nutrients.

Employ Icehack to enhance recovery

Icehack can help you feel your best and stay on track with your fitness objectives by reducing muscular discomfort after a workout.

Take Icehack with you everywhere you go

Icehack is available in easy-to-add-to-water-bottles on-the-go packages that make it simple to keep energised and focused all day long.

Conclusion

You may boost your weight loss efforts and enhance your general health by including Icehack into your routine. You can enhance weight reduction outcomes and meet your health objectives by using Icehack as a complement to a good diet and exercise plan. You may feel your best and lead a healthy, active lifestyle by introducing Icehack into your everyday routine with a little creativity and forethought.

Potential Challenges and How to Overcome Them

While adding Icehack into your lifestyle can have a variety of positive effects, it's crucial to be aware of any difficulties or roadblocks that might appear. In this part, we'll look at some typical problems that come up when using Icehack to lose weight and offer advice and solutions.

- **Icehack's flavor and texture may not be to everyone's liking or make eating it challenging.** To get past this obstacle, try combining Icehack with your preferred beverage or incorporating it into smoothies or energy bars.

- **Digestive issues:** Icehack may cause digestive issues for some individuals, such as bloating, gas, or upset stomach. To reduce the risk of digestive issues, start with a small dose of Icehack and gradually increase over time. It is also important to consume plenty of water and other hydrating fluids when using Icehack.

- **Cost:** Icehack may be more expensive than other supplements or weight loss products on the market. To overcome this challenge, consider buying in bulk or looking for discounts or promotions. You can also reduce the cost by using Icehack as a supplement to a healthy diet and exercise routine, rather than relying on it as the sole means of weight loss.

- **Convenience and time:** Including Icehack in your everyday routine could take more time and effort. Choose pre-packaged Icehack supplies that are convenient to take with you or prepare your Icehack in advance to get around this obstacle.

- **Plateaus and lack of results:** Some people who use Icehack may not experience the anticipated weight reduction outcomes or may hit a weight loss plateau. Consider speaking with a qualified dietician or healthcare expert to create a personalized plan that takes into consideration your unique requirements and health status in order to conquer this difficulty. To maintain a calorie deficit and maximize your weight reduction outcomes, it may also be beneficial to modify your workout regimen or eating habits.

Conclusion

While adding Icehack into your lifestyle can have a variety of positive effects, it's crucial to be aware of any difficulties or roadblocks that might appear. You may overcome these obstacles and maintain your weight loss goals by using the advice and methods provided in this section. Keep in mind that losing weight is a journey that calls for endurance, patience, and a comprehensive strategy that takes into account lifestyle, exercise, and food aspects. You can maximize weight loss outcomes and meet your health objectives by including Icehack into a healthy, balanced lifestyle.

Chapter 8

Other Health Benefits of Icehack

Despite the fact that Icehack is largely promoted as a weight-loss product, it also has a number of other health advantages that can help with overall wellbeing. We shall examine a few of Icehack's additional health advantages in this chapter which includes;

- **Increased cognitive function:** Caffeine, which is present in Icehack, can support increased mental clarity, attention, and alertness. Amino acids and other substances that can promote brain health and cognitive function are also included in Icehack.

- **Improved energy:** The natural stimulants found in Icehack, including caffeine, can help increase energy and lessen exhaustion. Athletes, students, and anyone else who needs to remain alert and focused throughout the day may find this to be very helpful.

- **Improved athletic performance**: It has been demonstrated that Icehack improves athletic performance by boosting endurance, cutting down on tiredness, and enhancing muscle function. Athletes or people who regularly engage in physical activity may find this to be particularly advantageous.

- **Decreased inflammation:** The anti-inflammatory substances included in Icehack can aid in reducing inflammation throughout the body. This is advantageous for everyone trying to lessen inflammation and promote general health, including those with inflammatory diseases like arthritis.

- **Enhanced cardiovascular health:** According to some research, Icehack may offer advantages for cardiovascular health, including lowering the risk of cardiovascular disease and raising cholesterol levels. These advantages might result from Icehack's anti-inflammatory and antioxidant qualities.

Enhanced gut health: The ingredients in Icehack have the ability to improve gut health by encouraging the growth of probiotics and lowering digestive tract inflammation.

Chapter 9

Conclusion and Final Thoughts

We have discussed the usage of Icehack as a supplement for weight loss and general health in this book. The science of weight loss, tracking and maintaining a calorie deficit, the importance of exercise and nutrition, and the drawbacks and advantages of utilizing Icehack have all been discussed.

Although Icehack can be a useful weight reduction tool, it's vital to keep in mind that lasting weight loss calls for a holistic strategy that include a good diet, consistent exercise, and a supportive lifestyle.

While Icehack can support these efforts, it shouldn't be used as a weight loss substitute.

When using Icehack to aid in weight reduction, it's crucial to adhere to the dosage guidelines and seek advice from a doctor or trained nutritionist if you have any worries about your health or if you have any pre-existing issues.

In addition to helping people lose weight, Icehack has a number of additional health advantages, including as higher physical performance, increased energy levels, improved cognitive function, and lower inflammation.

In general, Icehack can be a useful tool for people who want to support their overall health and weight loss goals. You may optimize Icehack's benefits and meet your health and wellness objectives by including it into a balanced, healthy lifestyle.

Future Developments in Icehack Research and Its Potential Impact on Weight Loss

Like with any dietary supplement, research on Icehack's benefits is continuing, and any new findings could have a significant impact on how well people lose weight and maintain general health. In terms of Icehack and weight loss, the following areas of research appear to be particularly promising:

- **Gut microbiome**: The gut microbiome is crucial for controlling weight, and some evidence indicates that Icehack may be beneficial for gut health. Icehack may become a more important tool for promoting gut health and weight loss as more is understood about the connection between the gut microbiome and weight loss.

- **The body's capacity to burn calories, or thermogenesis**, has been demonstrated to be increased by Icehack. Future studies could examine how Icehack affects the body's metabolic functions and how

- **Hormone balance:** Research suggests that Icehack may have a favorable effect on hormone balance, which is important for weight management. Icehack may be a useful technique for promoting hormonal balance and weight loss as more is understood about the connection between hormones and weight loss.

- **Individual differences**: Not everyone reacts to supplements in the same way, and some research indicates that hereditary variables may contribute to how people react to Icehack. As access to genetic testing and tailored nutrition increases, it might be able to customize Icehack supplementation to meet unique needs and maximize its impact on weight loss.

Overall, the ongoing research on Icehack and its effects on weight loss and overall health is promising. As more is learned about the mechanisms by which Icehack works, and how it interacts with other factors that influence weight management, its potential impact on weight loss may become even more significant.